CONTROVERSY AND CONTAGION: NAVIGATING THE MEASLES OUTBREAK

Insights into the Florida Epidemic and the Public Health Policy Struggle Amid Rising Infectious Threats

Dr. Sarah Willith

Table of Contents

Introduction

The Resurgence of Measles

Measles, once thought to be under control in many parts of the world, has experienced a troubling resurgence in recent years, challenging public health systems and raising concerns among medical professionals and policymakers alike. This chapter explores the factors contributing to the resurgence of measles, the global landscape of the disease, and the implications for public health.

The Historical Context

Measles, caused by the measles virus, has been a human affliction for centuries. Historically, outbreaks of measles were common, particularly in densely populated areas where the virus could spread rapidly among susceptible individuals. Before the introduction of vaccines, measles was a leading cause of childhood mortality worldwide.

In the 20th century, the development and widespread use of measles vaccines revolutionized public health efforts to control the disease. Vaccination campaigns led to a dramatic decline in measles cases and deaths, particularly in high-income countries where immunization programs were robust. At its peak, measles vaccination was hailed as one of the most successful public health interventions in history.

The Era of Decline and Elimination Efforts

By the turn of the 21st century, many regions had made significant progress towards measles elimination. The Americas, for example, declared measles eliminated in 2002, meaning that the virus no longer circulated continuously within the region. Similar efforts were underway in other parts of the world, with the goal of achieving measles elimination or eradication.

The success of measles control efforts was attributed to high vaccination coverage rates, which established herd immunity and reduced the pool of susceptible individuals. Herd immunity occurs when a significant proportion of the population is immune to a disease, thereby providing indirect protection to those who are not immune, including individuals who cannot be vaccinated for medical reasons.

The Resurgence Begins

However, despite decades of progress, the resurgence of measles has emerged as a significant public health challenge in recent years. Several factors have contributed to this resurgence, including:

1. **Declining Vaccination Rates**: In some communities, vaccination rates have fallen below the threshold needed to maintain herd immunity. This decline is often driven by misinformation and vaccine hesitancy, fueled by anti-vaccine movements and the spread of misinformation through social media and other channels.

Clinical Manifestations

Measles is caused by the measles virus, a member of the Paramyxoviridae family. The virus primarily targets the respiratory epithelium and lymphoid tissues, leading to a systemic infection characterized by a distinctive rash and a constellation of clinical symptoms.

The incubation period of measles is typically 10 to 14 days following exposure to the virus. The initial symptoms, often mistaken for a common cold, include high fever, cough, coryza (runny nose), and conjunctivitis (red, watery eyes). These prodromal symptoms precede the characteristic maculopapular rash, which typically appears 2 to 4 days after the onset of fever.

The measles rash typically begins on the face and behind the ears before spreading downward to the trunk and extremities. The rash is accompanied by fever spikes and may be associated with complications such as pneumonia, otitis media, encephalitis, and, in severe cases, death.

Modes of Transmission

Measles is highly contagious and spreads through respiratory droplets generated by coughing, sneezing, or talking. Infected individuals can transmit the virus to others from 4 days before to 4 days after the onset of the rash, making early identification and isolation crucial for preventing transmission.

Measles transmission occurs most commonly in settings where individuals are in close contact with one another, such as households, schools, childcare facilities, and healthcare settings. Crowded and poorly ventilated environments facilitate the spread of the virus, increasing the risk of outbreaks in susceptible populations.

The virus can survive in the environment for several hours, posing a risk of indirect transmission through contaminated surfaces and fomites. Vaccination remains the most effective means of preventing measles transmission, as it confers immunity to the virus and contributes to herd immunity within populations.

The Global Burden of Measles

Despite significant progress in measles control and elimination efforts, measles remains a major public health concern, particularly in regions with low vaccination coverage and limited access to healthcare services. According to the World Health Organization (WHO), measles continues to be a leading cause of vaccine-preventable deaths among children worldwide.

Outbreaks of measles continue to occur in various parts of the world, fueled by factors such as suboptimal vaccination coverage, population mobility, and vaccine hesitancy. In recent years, several countries have experienced large-scale measles outbreaks, underscoring the importance of maintaining high vaccination coverage rates and strengthening surveillance and response systems.

Conclusion

Measles is more than just a viral illness; it is a reminder of the enduring challenges of infectious disease control and the importance of vaccination in protecting public health. Understanding the historical, clinical, and epidemiological aspects of measles is essential for developing effective strategies for prevention, control, and ultimately, the eradication of this ancient scourge. In the chapters that follow, we will explore the intricacies of measles outbreaks, examine vaccination policies and strategies, and discuss the broader implications of measles resurgence in the 21st century.

Chapter 2 - The Florida Outbreak

Origins and Spread

The recent measles outbreak in Florida has raised significant concerns among public health officials, medical professionals, and the general population. This chapter aims to explore the origins of the outbreak, its spread within the state, and the factors contributing to its escalation.

Origins of the Outbreak

The Florida outbreak originated in Broward County, with the first cases identified in Manatee Bay Elementary School located in Weston, near Fort Lauderdale. The index case, or the first documented case, likely resulted from importation of the virus from outside the United States, as measles outbreaks often stem from travelers returning from regions with ongoing transmission or from exposure to international visitors.

The exact source of the index case may be challenging to determine, as measles is highly contagious and can spread rapidly within susceptible populations. However, investigations into the outbreak's origins typically involve contact tracing, genomic sequencing of the virus, and epidemiological analysis to identify potential sources of transmission.

In the case of the Florida outbreak, the spread of measles beyond the initial cluster of cases at Manatee Bay Elementary School suggests secondary transmission within the community. Measles can propagate quickly in settings where vaccination coverage is suboptimal, highlighting the importance of timely and targeted interventions to contain outbreaks.

Factors Contributing to Spread

Several factors contributed to the spread of measles within Florida and beyond:

1. **Suboptimal Vaccination Coverage**: Low vaccination coverage rates in certain communities create pockets of susceptibility where measles can gain a foothold and spread rapidly. Vaccine hesitancy, fueled by

misinformation and mistrust of vaccines, has led to declining immunization rates in some areas, increasing the risk of outbreaks.

2. **Crowded and Close Contact Settings**: Measles thrives in environments where individuals are in close proximity to one another, such as schools, daycare centers, and households. Crowded and poorly ventilated spaces facilitate transmission, making containment efforts challenging, particularly in densely populated urban areas.

3. **Challenges in Case Identification and Isolation**: The nonspecific nature of early measles symptoms, such as fever and cough, can make it difficult to identify cases early in the course of illness. Delayed

diagnosis and isolation of cases allow the virus to spread to others, amplifying the outbreak and complicating control efforts.

4. **Health Disparities and Access to Care**: Socioeconomic factors, including limited access to healthcare services and disparities in healthcare access, can exacerbate the impact of measles outbreaks, particularly among vulnerable populations. Addressing health inequities and ensuring equitable access to vaccines and healthcare are essential components of outbreak response strategies.

Response and Containment Efforts

In response to the measles outbreak, public health authorities in Florida implemented a range of containment measures aimed at preventing further transmission and protecting vulnerable populations. These efforts typically include:

- Enhanced surveillance and monitoring of suspected cases and contacts
- Promotion of measles vaccination through outreach and education campaigns
- Implementation of isolation and quarantine measures for individuals with suspected or confirmed measles
- Coordination with healthcare providers, schools, and community organizations to facilitate outbreak response and vaccination efforts

Lessons Learned and Future Considerations

The Florida measles outbreak underscores the ongoing threat posed by vaccine-preventable diseases and the importance of maintaining high vaccination coverage rates to prevent outbreaks and protect public health. Lessons learned from the outbreak can inform future efforts to strengthen vaccination programs, improve outbreak preparedness and response, and address underlying factors contributing to vaccine hesitancy and disparities in healthcare access.

In conclusion, the Florida measles outbreak serves as a stark reminder of the persistent challenges in infectious disease control and the critical role of vaccination in safeguarding public health. By addressing the root causes of vaccine hesitancy, promoting evidence-based vaccination policies, and fostering collaboration between public health agencies, healthcare providers, and communities, we can work towards preventing future outbreaks and ensuring the health and well-being of all individuals.

Chapter 3 - Controversies in Public Health Policy

The Role of Vaccination

Vaccination has long been heralded as one of the most effective public health interventions in human history, responsible for the eradication of deadly diseases and the prevention of countless illnesses and deaths worldwide. However, despite its undisputed success, vaccination remains a topic of controversy and debate in public health policy. This chapter explores the various controversies surrounding vaccination, including vaccine hesitancy, misinformation, ethical considerations, and the role of public health policy in promoting vaccination uptake.

Understanding Vaccine Hesitancy

Vaccine hesitancy refers to the delay in acceptance or refusal of vaccines despite the availability of vaccination services. It is a complex phenomenon influenced by a multitude of factors, including:

- **Safety Concerns**: Vaccine safety is a primary concern for many individuals and families. Misinformation and misconceptions about vaccine ingredients, side effects, and long-term health effects contribute to vaccine hesitancy and erode confidence in immunization programs.

- **Mistrust of Authorities**: Mistrust of government agencies, pharmaceutical companies, and healthcare providers can undermine confidence in vaccination recommendations. Historical injustices, such as unethical medical experimentation and breaches of trust, have fueled skepticism and reluctance to adhere to vaccination guidelines.

- **Cultural and Religious Beliefs**: Cultural and religious beliefs may shape attitudes towards vaccination, influencing decisions about vaccine acceptance and refusal. Some communities may have reservations about certain vaccines due to religious prohibitions or cultural practices, leading to disparities in vaccination coverage and susceptibility to vaccine-preventable diseases.

- **Social Media and Misinformation**: The proliferation of misinformation and anti-vaccine propaganda on social media platforms has contributed to vaccine hesitancy and vaccine refusal. False claims about vaccine safety, efficacy, and necessity can spread rapidly online, amplifying fears and undermining public confidence in vaccination.

Ethical Considerations in Vaccination Policy

Vaccination policy raises ethical considerations related to individual rights, public health, and social responsibility. Key ethical principles guiding vaccination policy include:

- **Beneficence**: Vaccination programs aim to promote the health and well-being of individuals and populations by preventing illness, reducing morbidity and mortality, and minimizing the burden of vaccine-preventable diseases.

- **Autonomy**: Individuals have the right to make informed decisions about their healthcare, including whether to accept or decline vaccination. Respect for individual autonomy requires transparent communication, informed consent processes, and efforts to address concerns and misinformation about vaccines.

- **Justice**: Vaccination policies should strive for equitable access to vaccines and healthcare services, particularly among marginalized and underserved populations. Efforts to reduce health disparities, address social determinants of health, and promote vaccine equity are integral to achieving health justice.

- **Public Health Utility**: Vaccination policies should prioritize the public health benefits of immunization, balancing individual rights with the collective responsibility to protect vulnerable populations and prevent the spread of infectious diseases.

Role of Public Health Policy

Public health policy plays a central role in promoting vaccination uptake, ensuring vaccine safety and efficacy, and addressing vaccine hesitancy and refusal. Key elements of effective vaccination policy include:

- **Vaccine Mandates**: Vaccine mandates require individuals to receive certain vaccinations as a condition of school enrollment, employment, or participation in certain activities. While controversial, vaccine mandates have been instrumental in increasing vaccination coverage and reducing the incidence of vaccine-preventable diseases.

- **School Immunization Requirements**: Many states and countries have implemented school immunization requirements to protect students, staff, and the community from vaccine-preventable diseases. These requirements typically specify the vaccines required for school entry and may include exemptions for medical, religious, or philosophical reasons.

- **Public Health Education and Communication**: Public health agencies play a crucial role in providing accurate, accessible, and culturally sensitive information about vaccines and vaccination. Educational campaigns, community outreach initiatives, and media engagement efforts can help counter misinformation, build trust, and promote vaccine acceptance.

- **Surveillance and Monitoring**: Robust surveillance systems are essential for monitoring vaccine-preventable diseases, detecting outbreaks, and assessing vaccination coverage and vaccine safety. Timely data collection, analysis, and dissemination inform policy decisions, guide resource allocation, and support outbreak response efforts.

Conclusion

Vaccination is a cornerstone of public health policy, saving lives and preventing suffering from infectious diseases. However, vaccine hesitancy, misinformation, and ethical considerations pose challenges to vaccination efforts and require comprehensive, evidence-based strategies to address. By promoting vaccine confidence, fostering trust in immunization programs, and prioritizing health equity and social justice, public health policy can help ensure the success of vaccination initiatives and protect the health of individuals and communities.

Chapter 4 - Inside Manatee Bay Elementary

A Case Study of Outbreak Management

The outbreak of measles at Manatee Bay Elementary School in Weston, Florida, serves as a compelling case study of the challenges and complexities involved in managing infectious disease outbreaks within educational settings. This chapter explores the timeline of the outbreak, the response efforts undertaken by public health authorities and school administrators, and the lessons learned from this experience.

Timeline of the Outbreak

The outbreak at Manatee Bay Elementary School unfolded over a period of several weeks, with multiple cases of measles identified among students, staff, and members of the surrounding community. The timeline of the outbreak can be broken down into several key phases:

1. **Initial Case Identification**: The outbreak began with the identification of the index case, or the first documented case of measles, within the school community. The index case likely resulted from exposure to the virus outside the school setting, highlighting the interconnectedness of communities and the potential for imported cases to trigger outbreaks.

2. **Rapid Transmission and Secondary Cases**: Following the identification of the index case, measles spread rapidly within the school environment, leading to secondary cases among students, staff, and family members. The highly contagious nature of measles, coupled with close contact within school settings, facilitated the transmission of the virus and fueled the outbreak's escalation.

3. **Community Impact and Public Health Response**: As the outbreak extended beyond the school campus, public health authorities in Broward County mobilized to contain the spread of measles and mitigate its impact on the community. Enhanced surveillance, contact tracing, and vaccination campaigns were implemented to

identify cases, isolate affected individuals, and prevent further transmission.

4. **Collaboration and Communication**: School administrators worked closely with public health officials to coordinate outbreak response efforts, communicate with parents and stakeholders, and implement infection control measures within the school environment. Transparent communication, timely updates, and collaboration between school and health authorities were critical components of the response strategy.

5. **Resolution and Lessons Learned**: Through concerted efforts to identify and isolate cases, promote vaccination, and educate the community about measles

prevention, the outbreak at Manatee Bay Elementary was eventually brought under control. However, the experience yielded valuable insights into the challenges of outbreak management and highlighted opportunities for improvement in preparedness, response, and communication strategies.

Response Efforts and Containment Measures

The response to the measles outbreak at Manatee Bay Elementary involved a multifaceted approach aimed at containing transmission, protecting vulnerable populations, and minimizing disruption to educational activities. Key response efforts included:

- Identification and Isolation of Cases: Prompt identification and isolation of individuals with suspected or confirmed cases of measles were essential for preventing further transmission within the school community. Students and staff exhibiting symptoms consistent with measles were advised to stay home, seek medical evaluation, and avoid contact with others until cleared by healthcare providers.

- Contact Tracing and Surveillance: Public health authorities conducted thorough contact tracing to identify individuals who may have been exposed to measles and assess their vaccination status and risk of infection. Close contacts of confirmed cases were monitored for symptoms and offered post-exposure prophylaxis or vaccination as appropriate.

- Vaccination Campaigns: Vaccination campaigns were launched to increase measles immunity among students, staff, and community members. Vaccine clinics were organized on-site at the school and in nearby neighborhoods to facilitate access to measles-containing vaccines and promote vaccine uptake among eligible individuals.

- Environmental Disinfection and Infection Control: Enhanced cleaning and disinfection protocols were implemented within the school environment to minimize the risk of environmental contamination and reduce the spread of measles virus particles. High-touch surfaces, common areas, and classroom facilities were regularly sanitized to maintain a safe and hygienic learning environment.

- Community Engagement and Education: School administrators and public health officials engaged with parents, students, and stakeholders to provide accurate information about measles, vaccination, and outbreak response efforts. Educational materials, informational sessions, and digital communications were utilized to address concerns, dispel myths, and encourage adherence to public health recommendations.

Lessons Learned and Best Practices

The measles outbreak at Manatee Bay Elementary highlighted several key lessons and best practices for managing infectious disease outbreaks within school settings:

1. Importance of Vaccination: Maintaining high vaccination coverage rates among students and staff is critical for preventing outbreaks and protecting vulnerable populations against vaccine-preventable diseases.

2. Early Detection and Response: Early detection of cases, coupled with rapid response and containment measures, can help limit the spread of infectious diseases and mitigate the impact of outbreaks on school communities.

3. Effective Communication and Collaboration: Transparent communication,

collaboration between school and health authorities, and engagement with parents and stakeholders are essential for building trust, promoting adherence to public health guidelines, and fostering a sense of community resilience during outbreaks.

4. Infection Control and Hygiene Practices: Implementing rigorous infection control measures, including hand hygiene, respiratory etiquette, and environmental disinfection, can help minimize the risk of disease transmission within school environments and promote a culture of health and safety.

5. Continuity of Education and Support Services: Maintaining continuity of education and support services for students

and families affected by outbreaks is paramount, requiring flexibility, creativity, and resourcefulness in adapting instructional delivery models and providing necessary accommodations and resources.

In conclusion, the measles outbreak at Manatee Bay Elementary serves as a poignant reminder of the ongoing threat posed by infectious diseases and the importance of proactive outbreak preparedness, effective response strategies, and collaborative partnerships in safeguarding the health and well-being of school communities. By applying lessons learned from this experience and embracing a culture of resilience, schools and public health authorities can strengthen their capacity to prevent and mitigate the impact of future outbreaks, ensuring a safe and supportive learning environment for all.

Chapter 5 - Measles and International Travel

Global Implications

Measles, a highly contagious viral infection, poses significant challenges to global health security, particularly in the context of international travel and mobility. This chapter examines the interplay between measles transmission and international travel, explores the factors contributing to the spread of measles across borders, and discusses the global implications of measles outbreaks in an interconnected world.

The Global Landscape of Measles

Measles remains endemic in many parts of the world, despite decades of vaccination efforts and progress towards measles elimination. While significant strides have been made in reducing measles-related morbidity and mortality, the persistence of measles transmission in certain regions underscores the ongoing threat posed by the virus.

Measles outbreaks continue to occur in both high-income and low-income countries, driven by a variety of factors, including:

1. Suboptimal Vaccination Coverage: Inadequate vaccination coverage rates, particularly among vulnerable populations, create pockets of susceptibility where

measles can gain a foothold and spread rapidly. Disparities in access to healthcare services, vaccine hesitancy, and logistical challenges in vaccine delivery contribute to suboptimal vaccination coverage in some communities.

2. Population Mobility and Migration: Population mobility, including international travel and migration, plays a significant role in the spread of measles across borders. Infected travelers can introduce the virus into susceptible populations, leading to outbreaks in regions with low vaccination coverage or waning immunity.

3. Conflict and Humanitarian Crises: Conflict-affected areas and regions experiencing humanitarian crises are

particularly susceptible to measles outbreaks due to disruptions in healthcare infrastructure, mass displacement of populations, and limited access to essential healthcare services, including vaccination.

4. Vaccine Supply Chain and Infrastructure Challenges: Weaknesses in vaccine supply chains, logistical constraints, and infrastructure challenges can impede the delivery of vaccines to remote or underserved areas, hindering efforts to achieve and maintain high vaccination coverage rates.

The Role of International Travel in Measles Transmission

International travel facilitates the spread of measles by enabling the movement of infected individuals across borders and continents. Measles is highly contagious, with transmission occurring through respiratory droplets generated by coughing, sneezing, or talking. Infected individuals can shed the virus and infect others during the prodromal phase of illness, before the characteristic rash appears.

Measles transmission on airplanes and other modes of transportation is well-documented, particularly in crowded and enclosed environments where close contact occurs. Infected travelers may unknowingly expose fellow passengers, crew members, and airport personnel to the virus, increasing the risk of secondary transmission and seeding new outbreaks in destination countries.

The incubation period of measles ranges from 7 to 21 days, allowing infected travelers to develop symptoms and become contagious after arriving at their destination. As a result, imported cases of measles can lead to localized outbreaks in communities with low vaccination coverage or pockets of susceptibility, amplifying the public health impact of international travel-related transmission.

Preventing Measles Transmission During Travel

Effective strategies for preventing measles transmission during travel include:

1. Vaccination: Vaccination remains the most effective means of preventing measles transmission and protecting travelers from

infection. The Measles, Mumps, and Rubella (MMR) vaccine is highly effective in conferring immunity to measles and is routinely recommended for international travelers, particularly those visiting regions with endemic or epidemic measles transmission.

2. Pre-Travel Health Consultation: Travelers should seek pre-travel health consultation with healthcare providers or travel medicine specialists to assess their vaccination status, review travel itinerary and risk factors, and receive personalized recommendations for preventive measures, including vaccination, malaria prophylaxis, and food and water safety precautions.

3. Awareness and Education: Travelers should be educated about the signs and symptoms of measles, including fever, cough, runny nose, and characteristic rash, and instructed to seek medical attention if symptoms develop during or after travel. Awareness campaigns and educational materials can help raise awareness about measles transmission and prevention among travelers.

4. Infection Control Measures: Infection control measures, including hand hygiene, respiratory etiquette, and environmental disinfection, should be practiced during travel to reduce the risk of exposure to infectious agents, including measles virus. Travelers should be encouraged to practice good hand hygiene, cover coughs and

sneezes, and avoid close contact with individuals who appear ill.

Global Implications and Collaborative Efforts

Measles outbreaks have far-reaching implications for global health security, underscoring the need for coordinated international efforts to prevent and control the spread of the virus. Key strategies for addressing measles transmission and mitigating its impact on global health include:

1. Enhancing Surveillance and Response Capacity: Strengthening surveillance systems, enhancing laboratory capacity, and improving outbreak detection and response capabilities are essential for early

identification and containment of measles outbreaks at the national and international levels.

2. Promoting Vaccination Equity and Access: Ensuring equitable access to vaccines and strengthening immunization programs are critical for achieving and sustaining high vaccination coverage rates globally. Efforts to address vaccine inequities, expand vaccine delivery channels, and overcome logistical barriers to vaccine access are essential for achieving measles elimination goals.

3. Fostering Multisectoral Collaboration: Collaboration between governments, international organizations, civil society, and the private sector is essential for

addressing the multifaceted challenges posed by measles transmission and promoting sustainable solutions for disease prevention and control.

4. Advocating for Vaccine Confidence and Public Trust: Building public trust in vaccines, addressing vaccine hesitancy, and countering misinformation are fundamental to sustaining public support for vaccination programs and achieving community immunity against measles and other vaccine-preventable diseases.

In conclusion, the intersection of measles and international travel underscores the interconnectedness of global health and the importance of collective action in addressing infectious disease threats. By promoting vaccination, strengthening health systems, and fostering international cooperation, the global community can work towards achieving measles elimination and ensuring a healthier and more resilient world for all.

Chapter 6 - The Battle Against Misinformation

Debunking Myths and Promoting Vaccination

In the fight against infectious diseases, vaccination stands as a cornerstone of public health. However, the effectiveness of vaccination programs is often challenged by misinformation, myths, and misconceptions surrounding vaccines. This chapter delves into the pervasive nature of vaccine misinformation, explores common myths and misconceptions, and outlines strategies for debunking myths and promoting vaccination to protect public health.

The Pervasiveness of Vaccine Misinformation

Misinformation about vaccines has proliferated in recent years, fueled by a myriad of sources including social media, online forums, celebrity endorsements, and alternative health practitioners. Vaccine misinformation can take various forms, ranging from outright falsehoods to subtle distortions of scientific evidence. Common myths and misconceptions about vaccines include:

1. Link Between Vaccines and Autism: One of the most enduring myths surrounding vaccines is the debunked claim that vaccines, particularly the measles, mumps, and rubella (MMR) vaccine, cause autism spectrum disorders. Despite numerous

scientific studies debunking this claim, it continues to persist in public discourse, perpetuating fears and vaccine hesitancy among parents.

2. Natural Immunity vs. Vaccination: Some individuals believe that natural immunity acquired through exposure to infectious diseases is superior to immunity conferred by vaccines. This misconception overlooks the risks associated with natural infection, including severe illness, complications, and death, and undermines the lifesaving benefits of vaccination.

3. Perceived Safety Concerns: Concerns about vaccine safety, including the presence of additives such as thimerosal and aluminum, have contributed to vaccine

hesitancy and refusal. While extensive scientific research has demonstrated the safety and efficacy of vaccines, perceptions of risk and mistrust of regulatory authorities continue to shape attitudes towards vaccination.

4. Herd Immunity and Vaccine Efficacy: Misunderstandings about herd immunity, the concept that high vaccination coverage rates within a population protect individuals who cannot be vaccinated, have led some individuals to question the necessity of vaccination. Skepticism about vaccine efficacy and the perceived insignificance of individual contributions to herd immunity undermine collective efforts to prevent disease transmission.

Debunking Vaccine Myths and Misconceptions

Addressing vaccine misinformation requires a multifaceted approach that combines scientific literacy, evidence-based communication, and community engagement. Key strategies for debunking vaccine myths and promoting vaccination include:

1. Education and Empowerment: Providing accurate, accessible, and culturally sensitive information about vaccines and vaccination is essential for empowering individuals and communities to make informed decisions about their health. Educational campaigns, public forums, and interactive resources can help dispel myths, address concerns, and build confidence in vaccination.

2. Fostering Trust and Credibility: Establishing trust and credibility with audiences is critical for effective communication about vaccines. Healthcare providers, public health officials, and trusted community leaders play pivotal roles in disseminating accurate information, addressing concerns, and countering misinformation through transparent and empathetic communication.

3. Engaging with Vaccine Hesitant Communities: Engaging directly with vaccine-hesitant communities and understanding the underlying reasons for vaccine hesitancy are essential for developing tailored interventions and building trust. Listening to concerns, acknowledging uncertainties, and

addressing misinformation in a nonjudgmental manner can help bridge communication gaps and foster meaningful dialogue.

4. Leveraging Social Media and Digital Platforms: Harnessing the power of social media and digital platforms to disseminate accurate information, counter misinformation, and amplify trusted sources is key to reaching diverse audiences and promoting vaccine acceptance. Digital literacy programs, fact-checking initiatives, and collaboration with social media influencers can help combat the spread of vaccine misinformation online.

5. Highlighting Personal Stories and Testimonials: Sharing personal stories and

testimonials from individuals who have experienced the devastating consequences of vaccine-preventable diseases can underscore the importance of vaccination and humanize the impact of misinformation. Personal narratives can resonate emotionally with audiences and inspire action to protect against vaccine-preventable diseases.

Promoting Vaccine Advocacy and Policy Support

Advocacy for vaccination and supportive policy measures are integral components of efforts to combat vaccine misinformation and promote vaccine acceptance. Key strategies for promoting vaccine advocacy and policy support include:

1. Advocating for Evidence-Based Policies: Advocacy efforts aimed at promoting evidence-based vaccination policies, including school immunization requirements, vaccine mandates, and public health campaigns, can help strengthen vaccination infrastructure and support public health objectives.

2. Collaborating with Stakeholders: Collaboration with government agencies, healthcare providers, advocacy organizations, and civil society groups is essential for advancing vaccine advocacy efforts and mobilizing support for vaccination programs. Collective action and partnerships can amplify advocacy messages, leverage resources, and drive policy change.

3. Legislative and Regulatory Initiatives: Supporting legislative and regulatory initiatives aimed at enhancing vaccine access, addressing vaccine misinformation, and strengthening immunization programs can help create an enabling environment for vaccination and safeguard public health.

4. Community Mobilization and Grassroots Advocacy: Empowering communities to advocate for vaccination through grassroots initiatives, community-led campaigns, and civic engagement efforts can foster a sense of ownership and commitment to vaccine advocacy goals. Building coalitions, organizing events, and mobilizing support at the local level can drive meaningful change and promote vaccine acceptance.

Conclusion

The battle against vaccine misinformation is a critical frontier in the fight to protect public health and prevent infectious diseases. By debunking myths, promoting accurate information, fostering trust, and advocating for evidence-based policies, we can confront vaccine hesitancy, strengthen immunization programs, and ensure a healthier and more resilient future for individuals and communities worldwide. Through collective action, education, and advocacy, we can overcome the challenges posed by vaccine misinformation and build a world where everyone has access to life-saving vaccines and the protection they provide against preventable diseases.

Chapter 7 - Confronting Legal and Ethical Dilemmas

Individual Rights vs. Public Health

In the realm of public health, the tension between individual rights and public health imperatives often gives rise to complex legal and ethical dilemmas. This chapter explores the intricate interplay between individual liberties and collective well-being, examines key legal and ethical principles guiding public health interventions, and navigates the challenges inherent in balancing competing interests in pursuit of the common good.

The Primacy of Public Health

Public health, as a field of practice and policy, is rooted in the principle of promoting and protecting the health of populations. From disease surveillance and outbreak response to vaccination programs and environmental regulations, public health initiatives are designed to safeguard the welfare of communities and prevent harm on a collective scale.

At the heart of public health endeavors lie core principles such as:

1. Prevention: Proactive measures aimed at preventing disease, injury, and disability before they occur form the cornerstone of public health practice. Strategies may include health education, immunization, screening, and policy interventions designed

to mitigate risk factors and promote healthy behaviors.

2. Equity: The pursuit of health equity underpins efforts to address health disparities and promote fair and just distribution of resources, opportunities, and outcomes across diverse populations. Equity considerations inform policies and programs aimed at reducing social determinants of health and addressing systemic barriers to health access and opportunity.

3. Community Engagement: Meaningful engagement with communities, stakeholders, and affected populations is essential for building trust, fostering collaboration, and ensuring that public

health interventions are culturally responsive, contextually appropriate, and responsive to community needs and priorities.

Legal Frameworks and Public Health Powers

In the United States and other jurisdictions, public health authorities possess broad legal powers to protect and promote the health of populations. These powers, derived from constitutional provisions, statutes, regulations, and case law, grant public health agencies the authority to enact and enforce a wide range of measures, including:

1. Quarantine and Isolation: Public health authorities may impose quarantine and isolation orders to prevent the spread of

contagious diseases and protect the public from exposure to infectious agents. Quarantine involves the restriction of movement for individuals who have been exposed to a contagious disease but are not yet symptomatic, while isolation applies to individuals who are known or suspected to be infected and pose a risk of transmission to others.

2. Mandatory Vaccination: Vaccination mandates, requiring individuals to receive certain vaccines as a condition of school enrollment, employment, or participation in certain activities, are a common public health intervention aimed at achieving herd immunity and preventing outbreaks of vaccine-preventable diseases. While vaccination mandates have been upheld by

courts in many jurisdictions, they remain subject to legal challenges and controversy.

3.   Surveillance and Reporting Requirements: Public health agencies collect and analyze data on disease occurrence, morbidity, and mortality to monitor trends, detect outbreaks, and inform public health decision-making. Reporting requirements mandate healthcare providers, laboratories, and other entities to report specified diseases, conditions, and events to public health authorities for surveillance and response purposes.

4.   Environmental Regulations: Environmental health regulations, including air and water quality standards, food safety regulations, and occupational health

standards, aim to protect individuals and communities from environmental hazards and prevent adverse health outcomes associated with exposure to pollutants, toxins, and other harmful agents.

While public health powers are essential for safeguarding the common good and promoting population health, they can also raise significant legal and ethical questions regarding individual rights, autonomy, and due process.

Legal and Ethical Considerations

The exercise of public health powers often implicates fundamental rights and liberties guaranteed by constitutions, laws, and international agreements. Key legal and ethical considerations in navigating the tension between individual rights and public health include:

1. Proportionality and Necessity: Public health interventions should be proportionate to the public health threat they seek to address and grounded in scientific evidence, risk assessment, and consideration of less restrictive alternatives. Measures that infringe upon individual rights should be necessary, effective, and based on the best available evidence.

2. Least Restrictive Means: Public health measures should be implemented using the least restrictive means necessary to achieve their intended public health objectives. Efforts to protect public health should strive to minimize interference with individual

liberties and respect principles of least intrusion and minimal coercion.

3. Transparency and Accountability: Transparency in decision-making, clear communication of rationale and objectives, and meaningful engagement with affected individuals and communities are essential for building public trust, promoting accountability, and ensuring that public health interventions are grounded in principles of fairness, justice, and respect for human rights.

4. Due Process and Judicial Review: Individuals subject to public health interventions, such as quarantine orders or vaccination mandates, have the right to due process and judicial review to challenge the

legality and constitutionality of government actions. Judicial oversight serves as a safeguard against abuse of power, arbitrary decision-making, and violations of individual rights.

Navigating Legal and Ethical Dilemmas

Navigating the complex terrain of legal and ethical dilemmas in public health requires careful consideration of competing interests, values, and principles. Strategies for addressing legal and ethical dilemmas include:

1. Stakeholder Engagement: Engaging with stakeholders, including affected individuals, community representatives, advocacy groups, and legal experts, fosters dialogue,

builds consensus, and promotes accountability in decision-making processes.

2. Ethical Deliberation and Analysis: Ethical frameworks, such as principles of public health ethics, human rights, and bioethics, provide guidance for ethical deliberation, analysis, and decision-making in public health practice. Ethical impact assessments, stakeholder consultations, and deliberative processes can help identify and address ethical considerations in public health policy and practice.

3. Interdisciplinary Collaboration: Collaboration between public health professionals, legal experts, ethicists, policymakers, and community stakeholders

facilitates interdisciplinary dialogue, knowledge exchange, and creative problem-solving approaches to address complex legal and ethical dilemmas in public health.

4. Continuous Evaluation and Adaptation: Public health policies and interventions should be subject to continuous evaluation, monitoring, and adaptation in light

Chapter 8 - Lessons Learned and Strategies for the Future

In the ever-evolving landscape of public health, reflecting on lessons learned and identifying strategies for the future are essential for advancing the collective goal of promoting health and well-being for all. This chapter explores key lessons gleaned from past experiences, examines emerging challenges and opportunities, and outlines proactive strategies to address current and future public health priorities.

Lessons Learned

1.   Preparedness   and   Resilience: The COVID-19   pandemic   underscored   the importance of preparedness and resilience in   responding   to   global   health   crises. Investing   in   robust   public   health infrastructure,   surveillance   systems,   and emergency response capabilities is essential for   mitigating   the   impact   of   infectious disease   outbreaks   and   other   health emergencies.

2. Equity and Social Determinants of Health: Health disparities magnified by the pandemic highlighted the urgent need to address underlying social determinants of health, including poverty, racism, and inequitable access to healthcare. Promoting health   equity   and   addressing   systemic

barriers to health access and opportunity are critical for achieving health justice and advancing health for all.

3. Interdisciplinary Collaboration: The complexity of public health challenges necessitates interdisciplinary collaboration and partnership across sectors, disciplines, and stakeholders. Building bridges between public health, healthcare, academia, government, industry, and civil society enhances synergy, fosters innovation, and amplifies collective impact in addressing shared health priorities.

4. Adaptive Leadership and Crisis Management: Adaptive leadership and effective crisis management are indispensable for navigating uncertainty,

complexity, and ambiguity in times of crisis. Leaders must demonstrate agility, empathy, and decisiveness in mobilizing resources, engaging stakeholders, and guiding response efforts to address evolving public health challenges.

5. Communication and Trust: Transparent communication, clear messaging, and trust-building are fundamental for fostering public trust, confidence, and compliance with public health recommendations. Building partnerships with communities, leveraging trusted messengers, and employing culturally sensitive communication strategies enhance credibility and promote shared responsibility for health.

Strategies for the Future

1. Investment in Public Health Infrastructure: Prioritizing investment in public health infrastructure, workforce development, and capacity-building is essential for strengthening pandemic preparedness, disease surveillance, and response capabilities. Sustainable funding mechanisms, strategic resource allocation, and interdisciplinary training programs enhance resilience and readiness for future health threats.

2. Health Equity and Social Justice: Advancing health equity and social justice requires a comprehensive approach that addresses structural inequities, dismantles systemic barriers, and promotes inclusive policies and programs. Targeted

interventions to address disparities in access to healthcare, housing, education, and employment empower marginalized communities and promote health equity for all.

3. Global Collaboration and Solidarity: The interconnected nature of global health demands collective action and solidarity across borders to address shared health challenges. Strengthening international cooperation, supporting multilateral institutions, and investing in global health security initiatives enhance preparedness, response, and resilience to emerging infectious diseases and other health threats.

4. Innovation and Technology: Harnessing innovation and technology holds promise

for transforming public health practice, improving healthcare delivery, and enhancing disease surveillance and monitoring. Embracing digital health solutions, artificial intelligence, genomics, and telemedicine expands access to care, facilitates data-driven decision-making, and accelerates progress towards health equity and sustainability.

5. Community Engagement and Empowerment: Empowering communities as active participants in the design, implementation, and evaluation of public health interventions fosters ownership, resilience, and sustainability. Community-driven approaches, participatory research methods, and culturally competent programming amplify

voices, address local priorities, and promote collective action for health and well-being.

6. Education and Health Literacy: Investing in health education, promotion, and literacy equips individuals and communities with knowledge, skills, and resources to make informed decisions and adopt healthy behaviors. Lifelong learning opportunities, school-based health education, and digital health literacy initiatives enhance health literacy and empower individuals to navigate complex health information landscapes.

7. Policy Advocacy and Governance: Advocating for evidence-based policies, legislation, and regulations that promote health and well-being is essential for

shaping environments, systems, and behaviors conducive to health. Civil society engagement, policy advocacy campaigns, and governance reforms strengthen accountability, transparency, and participatory decision-making in public health governance.

Conclusion

As we reflect on past experiences and look towards the future, the lessons learned from the COVID-19 pandemic and other public health challenges underscore the importance of resilience, collaboration, and innovation in advancing health and well-being for all. By embracing a holistic approach to public health, grounded in equity, solidarity, and community empowerment, we can navigate the complexities of our rapidly changing world and build a healthier, more resilient future for generations to come. Through shared vision, collective action, and unwavering commitment to the common good, we can turn challenges into opportunities and shape a brighter tomorrow for global health.

Chapter 9 - Conclusion

Towards a Measles-Free Future

Measles, once considered a disease of the past, continues to pose significant threats to global health and well-being. Despite the availability of safe and effective vaccines, measles outbreaks persist, fueled by gaps in vaccination coverage, vaccine hesitancy, and systemic challenges in disease control efforts. As we reflect on the lessons learned, challenges faced, and progress made in the battle against measles, it becomes increasingly clear that concerted action and unwavering commitment are needed to achieve a measles-free future.

The Persistent Threat of Measles

Measles, caused by the highly contagious measles virus, remains a leading cause of vaccine-preventable morbidity and mortality worldwide. The resurgence of measles outbreaks in recent years underscores the persistent threat posed by the virus, particularly in regions with suboptimal vaccination coverage and weak health systems. The consequences of measles extend beyond individual health outcomes, encompassing economic burdens, healthcare strain, and societal disruption.

Lessons Learned from the Past

The fight against measles has yielded valuable lessons that inform our approach to disease control and prevention. From the successful eradication of endemic measles in several regions to the challenges encountered in sustaining progress, our experiences have underscored the importance of:

1. Vaccination as a Cornerstone of Disease Control: Vaccination remains the most effective tool for preventing measles transmission and achieving population immunity. High vaccination coverage rates, coupled with robust immunization programs and surveillance systems, are critical for preventing outbreaks and protecting vulnerable populations.

2. Addressing Vaccine Hesitancy and Misinformation: Vaccine hesitancy and misinformation pose significant barriers to achieving vaccination goals and eradicating

measles. Strategies to address vaccine hesitancy include transparent communication, community engagement, and targeted interventions to counter misinformation and build trust in vaccines.

3. Equity in Access to Vaccines and Healthcare: Achieving health equity is essential for ensuring that all individuals have access to life-saving vaccines and essential healthcare services. Efforts to address disparities in access, address social determinants of health, and promote inclusive policies are integral to achieving measles elimination and advancing health equity for all.

4. Collaboration and Solidarity: Collaboration between governments,

international organizations, civil society, and the private sector is essential for coordinating efforts, mobilizing resources, and driving progress towards measles elimination goals. Global solidarity and shared responsibility are crucial for addressing cross-border challenges and achieving collective health outcomes.

Challenges and Opportunities Ahead

While progress has been made in reducing measles-related morbidity and mortality, significant challenges lie ahead on the path to measles elimination. Persistent gaps in vaccination coverage, outbreaks fueled by vaccine misinformation, and logistical challenges in vaccine delivery underscore the need for sustained commitment, innovation, and investment in disease control efforts. However, amidst these challenges, there are also opportunities to strengthen our resolve, leverage new technologies, and forge partnerships to accelerate progress towards a measles-free future.

Towards a Measles-Free Future
Achieving a measles-free future requires a multifaceted approach that integrates vaccination strategies, strengthens health systems, and addresses underlying determinants of disease transmission. Key components of our journey towards measles elimination include:

1. Enhancing Vaccination Coverage and Access: Scaling up vaccination coverage, reaching underserved populations, and

expanding access to vaccines are critical for achieving and sustaining measles elimination goals. Targeted vaccination campaigns, innovative delivery models, and partnerships with communities and healthcare providers can help bridge gaps in coverage and reach vulnerable populations.

2. Investing in Surveillance and Response Capacity: Strengthening disease surveillance systems, enhancing laboratory capacity, and improving outbreak detection and response capabilities are essential for early identification and containment of measles outbreaks. Timely data collection, analysis, and dissemination enable rapid response efforts and informed decision-making in disease control initiatives.

3. Combatting Vaccine Misinformation and Hesitancy: Addressing vaccine misinformation, fostering vaccine confidence, and promoting evidence-based communication are integral to overcoming barriers to vaccination and achieving public trust in immunization programs. Education, advocacy, and collaboration with trusted messengers can help dispel myths, build resilience, and foster a culture of vaccine acceptance.

4. Advancing Health Equity and Social Justice: Prioritizing health equity, addressing disparities in access to healthcare, and addressing social determinants of health are essential for achieving measles elimination and promoting health equity for all. Policies and

programs that prioritize the needs of marginalized communities, promote inclusive decision-making, and address structural inequities are crucial for building a more just and equitable society.

5. Sustaining Global Commitment and Collaboration: Sustaining global commitment and collaboration is essential for achieving measles elimination goals and advancing global health security. Multilateral partnerships, resource mobilization efforts, and political will are vital for driving progress and overcoming barriers to measles eradication.

In conclusion, the journey towards a measles-free future is both a testament to human ingenuity and a call to action for collective responsibility. By harnessing the power of science, innovation, and solidarity, we can overcome the challenges posed by measles and create a world where every individual has the opportunity to live a healthy and fulfilling life, free from the threat of vaccine-preventable diseases. As we embark on this journey, let us remain steadfast in our commitment, unwavering in our resolve, and united in our pursuit of a brighter, healthier future for generations to come.